No White at Night

The Three Rule Diet

William A. Gavin, M.D.

First Edition 2003

Published by:
Eld Inlet Publishing, LLC
2103 Harrison NW, Suite 2 - 316
Olympia, WA 98502-2607
(360) 866-9401

Web Site: www.nowhiteatnight.com

First Printing 2003

ISBN 0-9741439-0-1
Library of Congress Controll Number: 2003093614

Dedication

To my parents for their love and guidance;

To my wife for her love and encouragement;

To my children for making me look like a good father.

CONTENTS

INTRODUCTION

You probably bought this book because you or a loved one is overweight. Congratulations, you have taken the first step towards managing the problem. In this book I will review the causes of obesity and outline several simple steps you can take towards overcoming your weight problem. It will not be easy, but once you understand the reasons why people gain weight, you will find it is not that hard to lose weight.

There is no simple pill or injection to cure obesity. There are usually multiple causes for an individual to gain weight and they will all need to be addressed. You will not learn *a diet* as you read this book. You will, however, learn a healthy approach to eating and exercise. The good news is that my patients who have achieved success through this approach, routinely come back and tell me, "It is not that hard."

This book in part has been a personal journey for me as well. If you were to look at me now, you would find it hard to believe that I ever had a weight problem. My current height is 6'1" and my weight is 167 pounds. I weighed approximately ten pounds less and was at least one foot shorter when I was in seventh grade. I was able to get my weight under control before I entered high school, and I did not really have a weight problem again until I was about thirty-five years old. From the age of thirty-five, I relentlessly gained 3-5 pounds per year. Finally, when I reached a weight of 210 pounds, I decided that was enough. It was time to lose weight. Some of the initial approaches I used to lose weight failed, but ultimately I achieved success. As I lost weight, I realized I had significant misconceptions about exercise and diet and the role they played in weight loss. So, I have come to understand what it means to be overweight and how challenging it can be to face up to the task of losing weight.

In my professional life as a cardiologist, I have seen the number of obese patients with various types of cardiovascular disease dramatically increase. In my office, on any given day, I usually counsel up to 30% or more of my patients about weight loss and diet. Initially, I recommended various programs such as Weight Watchers or books such as *The Zone Diet*[1]. What I found was both surprising and challenging.

Patients came back to my office saying they could not understand the various books they had purchased, they did not want to have to go to specific group meetings, and the multiple different types of diets and various guidelines available in the public media confused them. My patients did not understand the differences between the diets and subsequently they really could not then determine which one was right for them. The difficulties experienced by my patients reminded me of my own shortcomings in understanding my prior diet and exercise pattern. It occurred to me that I had a lot more training in nutrition and physiology than my patients did, therefore, if I had significant misconceptions at the start of my weight loss program, I really should not be surprised that my patients were having difficulty as well.

I discovered two important points about my patients in this process. My patients wanted their weight loss program to be simple: they did not want to have to weigh their individual food portions, they did not want to buy special foods, they did not want to make recipes from unfamiliar cookbooks, and they did not want to attend special meetings. The other point I discovered was how successful my patients could be in approaching weight loss if they understood the process. Whenever I could help my patients understand what the elements were that had caused them to gain weight, and how those elements could be individually changed, they had a significant improvement in weight loss success. So, I distilled down the important concepts of various diet programs and began recommending the principles defined in this book. These principles worked for the majority of my patients and I believe they will work for you too. We will take a detailed look at these principles later in the book.

First though, before we go through the principles, we need to review the role of a number of factors such as exercise, genetics and the role various food groups play in your diet. My reason for putting these chapters early in the book is to help you better understand the causes of obesity. Only after you understand the causes of obesity can you adequately address them in the long term.

As a physician, I have some misgivings about the validity of my approach. In medicine, new treatments are often subjected to large, randomized trials involving thousands of patients. In this type of study, some patients are treated and others serve as controls. It is a good approach and the fundamental basis for scientific evaluation in medicine. Unfortunately, this type of study has not been done for my diet principles or on a controlled basis between many of the popular diets that are currently available to the public. I would welcome anyone to fund such a trial.

As the problem of obesity gains more attention in the medical community, I suspect the government will ultimately fund patient treatment studies of this type. But even without a major study, I can say that my diet principles have been tested. These principles have been tested on myself with success. As I lost weight, my friends initially asked if I was okay. When I reassured them that my health was fine, they all wanted to know what I was doing to lose weight. So, after myself, these diet principles were tested on my friends, and then on my patients. I can now say I have hundreds of patients and friends who have been able to overcome their weight problems and significantly improve their health through weight loss. The success of these people and their encouragement led me to write this book. I believe this book can help you as well.

The challenge in writing this book is to transfer the experience that you would have as a patient in my office into these pages. If you visit with me in my office, I have the ability to explain concepts, and more importantly, answer your questions. The advantage to the book is that there is more time to explain the important concepts of obesity, exercise, and weight loss. The down side is that I cannot answer your specific questions directly. In counseling hundreds of patients over the last few years, I have come to understand the most common questions and have tried to address them in this book. When a patient leaves my office, they have a copy of my three rules, but I also make sure they have concrete options for all three meals that include foods they like. By the time you finish this book you should also know what you will have for breakfast, lunch and dinner on a routine basis.

There is an old Chinese proverb that a journey of a thousand miles starts with a single step. Your first step was to recognize that you or your loved one has a significant weight problem. Buying the book is another step. Reading this book alone will not allow you to lose weight. Reading this book and following the principles regarding diet and exercise will. As you read the book, think about when you started to gain weight or noticed that you had a weight problem. Think about what changed in your diet in the years prior to that. Start watching what you are eating, and especially start reading the labels of the foods that you are eating. Then you can begin to apply the principles of the book. You did not get overweight in a day and it will take you a considerable amount of time to lose your weight. You can lose the weight though, and you should enjoy the journey.

Chapter One
THE SUPERSIZING OF AMERICA

Americans young and old are getting fat. This medical fact has been discussed in the scientific literature for years and now is being actively covered in the popular press. In the past few months I have personally seen major stories on the obesity problem in the *Wall Street Journal*, *Newsweek*, and *Prevention* magazine. The government has even changed the tax code to allow deductions for monies paid towards weight loss therapies. The problem of obesity is now clearly on the radar screen of America and hopefully will be better addressed.

In 1980, the National Center for Health Statistics considered 46% of U.S. adults overweight or obese. Obesity is defined as being 20% above your ideal body weight. In 1999, the same group found that number had climbed to 60%[2]. The problem is not limited to adults. The CDC has declared obesity in children an epidemic. You really do not need to read the statistics to understand the magnitude of the problem. One only needs to look at the people in the supermarket or the public schools to see that a major problem exists.

The impact of obesity on your health is enormous.

Obesity is a major cause of high cholesterol (hypercholesterolemia or hyperlipidemia), diabetes mellitus and hypertension. These three illnesses are recognized risk factors for cardiovascular disease. Cardiovascular disease is the leading cause of death in the United States and most western industrialized countries. For this reason, the Surgeon General has declared that obesity now ranks only behind smoking as the health factor contributing to the greatest number of premature deaths in the United States.

The impact of obesity extends far beyond cardiovascular disease. Patient's suffering from obesity are more likely to suffer from arthritis; they are more likely to require joint replacements, or suffer disabling back injuries. Obesity prevents the early detection of problems such as breast cancer or abdominal aortic aneurysm. Both of these illnesses can have fatal consequences if not detected early. Thus, obesity can contribute to both premature death and disability. To help put it in quantifiable terms for the American public, a recent study in the *Journal of the American Medical Association* found that obese individuals had a significant reduction in life expectancy[3]. To use the example of young, white males who are obese, their life expectancy was shortened on average by thirteen years.

Ironically, many people do seem to understand they have a weight problem and try to address it. Americans are preoccupied with dieting and exercise. At any given time, 44% of women and 29% of men are said to be dieting[4]. The United States leads the world in the number of health clubs. So one needs to ask why Americans are having such poor outcomes in addressing their weight control problem.

The causes of the obesity epidemic are probably multifactorial. As we have become a more technologically oriented society, we have also become a more sedentary society. A decreased energy expenditure on a daily basis without any change in diet will lead to a slow, progressive weight gain. Decreased energy expenditure is not the only cause of the obesity problem, otherwise, exercise programs would resolve the issue. The fact is, most Americans are eating too many calories.

Food is plentiful and inexpensive in America. The USDA and other dietary advisor groups have recommended that Americans consume low-fat foods and these groups appear to have had significant success in getting their message to the American people. Most patients I see who are overweight do not consume high fat foods. My patients predominantly have a sedentary lifestyle and they consume an excessive amount of high calorie, low-fat carbohydrates. Unfortunately, many people believe that they can consume unlimited quantities of low-fat foods such as pasta or potatoes. You *can* get fat eating low-fat foods in unlimited quantities.

In summary, America has a major problem with obesity. The cause of the problem is multifactorial. Unfortunately, the solutions adopted by the average American in their diet and exercise pattern are not successful, at least over the long term. Before we review the potential solutions through diet and exercise, there are still some further issues that I think need to be reviewed as contributors to the obesity problem.

13

Chapter Two
EVOLUTION AND GENETICS

Nature has given us the ability to store calories as body fat. As noted earlier, obesity is now a major health risk. You may wonder why we need to be able to accumulate body fat. The simplest answer to the question is that nature has given us a tool for survival.

Throughout the thousands of years that humans have evolved, mankind has faced a major threat — famine. We happen to live in a unique time and place in history. Food is plentiful in the United States, but it was not always. Over 50% of the the early Jamestown colonists starved to death in their second year of settlement. In many parts of the world today, famine is still a major cause of death. In Southern Africa over the last year, the UN recognized that 16 million people were threatened by famine[5]. The unique combination of floods and drought as well as a failure by the government to adequately import maize contributed to the worst food shortage in a decade. Worldwide the number of people at risk for famine is considerably greater in any given year. To help us survive these times of food deprivation, it is necessary to have stored energy. In the human body, energy is predominantly stored as fat.

The ability to store fat may have also played a role in insuring survival of the species through reproduction. Women in general have a higher percentage of body fat than men. That is important for a woman's ability to carry a pregnancy to term and to nurse a newborn. Women who are malnourished stop menstruating and therefore lose the ability to reproduce. Thus, nature has probably given us the ability to store body fat to enable us to survive famine and also help insure propagation of the species. The biochemical processes, which determine our ability to store body fat, are in our genetic code.

All the biochemical reactions that occur in the body are determined by our individual genetic make-up. Half of your genes or chromosomes come from your mother and the other half from your father. I believe that the ability to store body fat is a genetic trait. Some people have a stronger ability to store fat than others. If you want to know if you have a tendency to get fat, look at your parents. I believe my own family is an excellent example.

My mother is a heavyset woman of German/Czech descent. My father is a thin Irishman. My mother has a very strong tendency to gain weight and has struggled with her weight over the years. My father has never had a weight problem over any significant period of time. My mother has tried various diet programs and actually achieved the most success through Weight Watchers. When I was a child, a typical story in the Gavin household was when my mother went on a diet my father would lose weight. Although you might think that my mother would be quite happy with my father's ability to remain thin, she actually became quite angry. When Mom was unhappy it was usually not an easy time for the men in the Gavin household. I would say that story played out at least every other year in the Gavin family.

My brothers and I are nearly a perfect example of mendelian genetic principles. There are five boys in the Gavin family. One brother looks like my mother, one brother looks like my father, three of the brothers are blends of our two parents. The brother who looks like my mother has a significant weight problem, and the brother who resembles my father always tended to be thin. The three blends have a tendency to vary their weight to the two greatest extremes. Personally, I am a blend.

Just as there seem to be people who are genetically more likely to gain weight through obesity, there are also people who never seem to gain weight. In our office we have one receptionist who is in her late 20's and is a mother. She is a true size 2. One day I sat down next to her at lunch and was amazed to see that she ate roughly twice as much as I did. Fortunately, she lives in a food plentiful society. If she or my father were in the Jamestown colony at the time of the famine, I doubt that either of them would have lived to see the springtime. I think my mother would have made it. Just as the United States is a very favorable place for people who do not have a very good ability to store body fat, it is a very hostile place for people who do have a strong tendency to gain weight, such as my mother or brother.

The important point in understanding how genetics affects obesity is to recognize that we are all unique individuals. Part of our individual variability is expressed in our tendency to store body fat. Simply having a predisposition to store body fat does not condemn you to being obese. It does, however, force you to be much more conscious of what you are eating and what impact the foods you consume have on your body weight. If you are an individual with a strong tendency towards obesity, that tendency will never go away. You were born with your genetic structure and it is with you for your entire life. For that reason you have to learn what foods are *right* for you and think about learning *how* to eat for a lifetime.

Chapter Three
EXERCISE

Everyone should have an exercise program. People who exercise often note an improved sense of well-being. Exercise will help lower your blood sugar, lower your blood pressure and raise your good cholesterol level. In contrast to obesity, the positive aspects of exercise will help lower your risk of cardiovascular disease. Personally I have tried to maintain some type of daily exercise pattern since I was in high school and I continue that to this day. What I have learned is that if you are overweight, it is not likely to be from lack of exercise alone.

Patients who come to see me and are overweight often believe the cause of their obesity is lack of exercise. I should point out that most of my patients are in their 40's or older. Sometimes my male patients have retired from physically demanding jobs in construction or the wood products industry. If you look at the calories that can be burned through exercise in Table 1, you note that it is hard to control your weight with exercise alone. To achieve weight loss of thirty pounds a year requires burning an excess 390 calories per day. As most of my patients are limited to walking as their predominant form of exercise, getting that

TABLE 1

Calories Expended for Various Activities*

Standing	104 cal./hr.
Walking - 2 mph	264 cal./hr.
Walking - 3 mph	352 cal./hr.
Walking - 4.5 mph	484 cal./hr.
Jogging - 5.5 mph	814 cal./hr.
Biking - 6 mph	264 cal./hr.
Biking - 12 mph	451 cal./hr.
Swimming - 25 yds./min.	302 cal./hr.
Jumping Rope	550 cal./hr.
Stair Master	300 - 600 cal./hr.
Eliptical Trainier	300 - 600 cal./hr.

*Based on 165 pound individual.

target of 390 calories daily would be very difficult. There is another reason I have come to believe that exercise alone will not lead to successful long-term weight loss: I've tried it. Let me tell you my personal experience.

When I had reached 210 pounds, I assumed I was overweight because I was not getting enough exercise. At that time I was exercising 4-5 days a week, usually on a Lifecycle exercise machine. I used that machine for at least thirty minutes every day I worked out. In spite of my exercise program, I found that my weight was going up relentlessly three to five pounds per year. I resolved that I would exercise more and started exercising seven days per week. I also rotated my exercise routine between the Lifecycle exercise bike and an elliptical trainer. The elliptical trainer is an exercise machine designed to mimic running but with a reduced knee and hip joint impact. The elliptical trainer has a higher calorie expenditure due to its similarity to running.

I lost ten pounds in the next six months through that change in exercise pattern. After that, my weight plateaued and I maintained that weight for an additional six months. At the end of the six months of being in a steady state, I changed my diet. Over the next fourteen months I lost thirty-five additional pounds. During the time I lost the additional weight, I kept my exercise pattern at the same higher level. But changing my diet combined with exercise gave me the most success. Bottom line, it is nearly impossible for the average patient to exercise their way out of a bad diet.

Another example of this principle is what I often over-hear when working out at our local health club. I work out alone, but a number of people get counseling from personal health trainers. A comment I have heard often is, "I've been doing this for two months now and haven't lost any weight." I think these people haven't yet made the realization that they have to change their diet as well as their exercise pattern to lose weight.

The illustration in Table 2 shows the dramatic effect of combining exercise with diet. I will make the assumption that the people in the health club frustrated with their lack of weight loss were motivated to initiate their exercise program to not only improve their fitness, but to lose weight. So let's say that they are on a diet and exercise program that led them to gain five pounds per year. If you change your exercise pattern to lose ten pounds per year, this is a significant and positive step. What the patient experiences though, is only a weight loss of five pounds per year as half of the weight loss of the improved exercise program is canceled by the weight gain mediated by their chronic diet pattern.

The dramatic effect of combining exercise and diet is shown in the second illustration in the table. If we take the same person who is gaining five pounds per year and change their diet to allow them to lose ten pounds per year through their diet alone, they will quadruple their overall weight loss. That person now is losing ten pounds a year through exercise and ten pounds per year through diet. The weight loss that can be achieved through exercise is

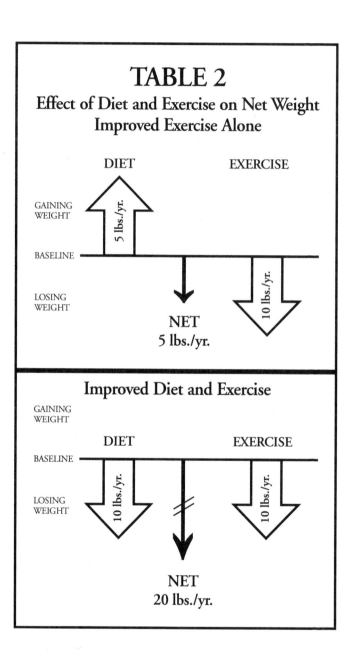

TABLE 2
Effect of Diet and Exercise on Net Weight
Improved Exercise Alone

DIET   EXERCISE

GAINING WEIGHT

5 lbs./yr.

BASELINE

LOSING WEIGHT

10 lbs./yr.

NET
5 lbs./yr.

Improved Diet and Exercise

GAINING WEIGHT

DIET   EXERCISE

BASELINE

LOSING WEIGHT

10 lbs./yr.   10 lbs./yr.

NET
20 lbs./yr.

markedly amplified through changing your diet.

As I said earlier, everyone should have an exercise program. Walking by itself is a great form of exercise. A recent study published in the *Journal of the American Medical Association*[6] looked at postmenopausal women and the impact of exercise on their weight. The predominant form of exercise was walking. These women lost between two and eight pounds per year. I think this is very realistic and applicable to the patients that I see in my practice all the time. For many of my arthritic or cardiac patients, walking is the only exercise they can do.

Recently the Institute of Medicine recommended that people get moderate physical activity for sixty minutes per day. This recommendation does not mean one hour of constant exercise. It can incorporate intermittent bursts of walking or stair climbing at work to total sixty minutes during the entire day. The Surgeon General has recommended thirty minutes of exercise per day since 1996.

I recommend to my patients that they walk at least thirty minutes per day. Whatever type of exercise you choose, make sure that it works for your individual schedule. I work out in the early morning because that is a predictable part of my day and I am unlikely to be called away to take care of patients. If you can get to an exercise facility, great, but if you cannot, try walking at work. Park ten minutes away from your work place if safety allows it, and then you will walk twenty minutes every day to and from work. Or take a walk on your lunch break. Whatever you choose for your exercise pattern, make it fit into your routine daily schedule so you can sustain it over the long term.

People vary in how they like to exercise. Some like to work out alone. Personally, I read the newspaper while riding on the exercise bike so I can kill two birds with one stone. Others choose exercise classes or prefer to walk with friends. There is no reason why you cannot integrate a social aspect into your exercise, especially if it helps you maintain your exercise regimen. Finally, if you do not think you are getting all the benefits you think you should with your exercise routine, ask a professional for help. Meet with a personal trainer, explain your goals, and develop a program that will work for you. Whatever you do, develop an exercise program.

Chapter Four
CALORIES IN, CALORIES OUT

We have now reviewed the role of exercise and genetics in the obesity problem. There is one more fundamental concept that people need to understand before we review many of the popular diets out in the public media. I refer to this concept as calories in versus calories out.

Your body is basically a reservoir. Every day you take in a number of calories and you expend a certain number of calories. If you take in more calories than you expend, the surplus calories are usually stored as body fat. If you expend more calories than you take in, you make up the extra calories needed usually by depleting your body fat. People can take in more calories by eating more food, especially if they eat energy rich foods high in sugar and fat. You can expend more calories through exercise. This concept is illustrated in Table 3.

Your body is a reservoir that reflects your net calorie intake and output over the years. It is no different than a reservoir of water that has streams flowing into it and streams flowing out of it. The water level will rise and fall based on inflow and outflow. If you bought this book with the goal of long-term weight loss, you need to stand in

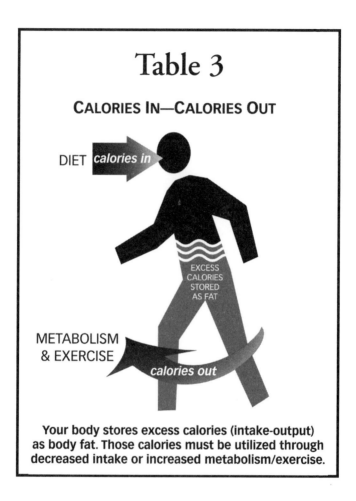

Table 3

CALORIES IN—CALORIES OUT

DIET *calories in*

EXCESS
CALORIES
STORED
AS FAT

METABOLISM
& EXERCISE

calories out

**Your body stores excess calories (intake-output)
as body fat. Those calories must be utilized through
decreased intake or increased metabolism/exercise.**

front of the mirror and recognize that your current body
weight is the result of your present diet and exercise pattern. You can change your diet, or your exercise pattern to
adjust your body fat, but failing to do this will not result
in any long-term sustained weight loss. As we noted in the

last chapter, weight loss can be achieved by either modulating diet or exercise. The greatest benefit, however, occurs if you change both diet and exercise. This is no different than in the reservoir analogy. The greatest change in the water level in the reservoir will occur if we decrease inflow and increase outflow.

It is unfortunate that many people hope there is some simple miracle pill out there that will cure their weight problem. It is even more disturbing to see advertisements frequently on TV or in the newspaper advocating some herbal or vitamin based cure that will melt your fat away while you sleep. There are medications such as amphetamines, or hormones such as thyroxine, that people can use for the purpose of weight loss. These drugs increase your metabolic rate, but with the risk of short and long term medical problems. There is no natural agent available in the marketplace that will turn your body into a thermonuclear reactor at night and melt away your body fat. As long as we are debunking myths, I will also tell you that there is no tooth fairy and Santa Claus did not leave your presents under the Christmas tree.

The long-term key to a successful weight control effort is through a combination of diet and exercise. The extra calories stored in your body are the result of overeating and must be burned off through calorie expenditure. Your body has been designed by nature to give up those calories only if it needs to. You cannot fight thousands of years of evolution. Once you accept that concept, it is much easier to move on.

Chapter Five
THE DIET SPECTRUM

The American public may be gaining weight and have an obesity problem but it is not for lack of popular diets available to them. There is a wide spectrum of diets available and each is considerably different. Which one is best is certainly becoming a topic of national prominence in part due to the obesity epidemic. I would like to put the different types of diets into perspective for you.

Most diets are referred to by name or a number ratio. Table 4 illustrates the spectrum of diets often touted as the best. When a diet is referred to by its individual components, it will have three percentages, such as 40-30-30. The first number is the percentage of total calories that come from carbohydrates. The second percentage is that of total calories from protein. The third number is the percent of total calories from fat. For example, in the American Heart Association diet, >55% of the total calories come from carbohydrate, <30% from protein and 15% from fat. The Zone Diet, in contrast, has 40% of its total calories from carbohydrate, roughly 30% from protein, and 30% from fat.

An important point to understand is the difference in

TABLE 4

Comparing low-carbohydrate diets with recommended diets

	Low Carbohydrate diets				Recommended Diets	
	Atkins	Protein Power	Sugar Busters	Zone	ADA* Exchange	AHA**
Total Daily calories (kcal)	1,600	1,600	1,600	1,600	1,600	1,600
Carbohydrates (g)	22 (5%)***	33 (8%)	162 (40%)	170 (40%)	240 (60%)	220 (>55%)
Protein (g)	146 (35%)	149 (35%)	113 (28%60	120 (28%)	82 (20%)	28-72 (12-18%)
Fat (g)	104 (59%)	97 (53%)	55 (32%)	49 (32%)	35 (20%)	53 (>30%)
Saturated fat (g)	47 (26%)	33 (19%)	17 (9%)	12 (7%)	11 (6%)	18 (<10%)
Cholesterol (mg)	924	657	280	264	112	<300
Dietary fiber (g)	4	11	24	18	22	>25

* ADA, American Diabetes Association.   ** AHA, American Heart Association   ***Percentage of total daily caloric intake.

Cleveland Clinic Journal of Medicine, Vol. 68, Sept. 2001

energy levels from the different food groups. Fat has the highest energy content at 9 calories per gram, carbohydrate at 5 calories per gram and protein at 4 calories per gram. Thus, even though the amount of fat and protein may be the same in a diet based on total caloric percentages, you would take in twice as much protein on a weight basis due to its lower energy content.

As you look at the various diets, there are some interesting comparisons. The first is that the amount of protein and fat as a percentage of total calories tends to be equal. The diets vary by their carbohydrate percentages. You might ask, "What is a low carbohydrate diet?" In the press and medical literature, low carbohydrate is defined as anything less than the carbohydrate content of the American Heart Association diet. I believe that is problematic because the Zone Diet, which is 40-30-30 is roughly 65% of the carbohydrate content of the American Heart Association diet but 400% of the carbohydrate content of the Atkin's diet. So what is low carbohydrate? There are a number of diets that exist in the 40-30-30 ratio. The Zone Diet may be the most well known, but also diets such as 40-30-30, Sugarbusters, Prism and Weight Watchers have somewhat similar calorie percentages.

My initial experiences in learning about these diets preceded my desire to counsel patients. I was interested at that time in losing weight myself. I initially started the process several years ago when I followed the American Heart Association diet and gained weight. I also gave up red meat and gained weight. What ultimately worked for me was moving from the percentages recommended by the American Heart Association Diet to the 40-30-30 area. I have maintained that nutritional balance and have not had any problems maintaining my weight over time.

The diet that is not addressed on the table is a vegetarian diet that actually has the highest percentage of carbohydrates at 80% of total calories. That is in part because it is hard to find protein sources without eating meat or fish that do not have high amounts of carbohydrate in them. Interestingly, I had noted for years that my patients who became vegetarians tended to gain weight. Initially, I found that perplexing, but now I understand the mechanism. Patients who are vegetarians have to consume a lot of carbohydrate to get adequate protein intake.

The observations I am going to make about the various diets are personal observations. I have not subjected these observations to randomized trials to prove them. I have, however, watched my patients for years and I can tell you what has worked for them and what has worked for myself as well. I will also note that I do not think there is an ideal diet for all patients. Patients are all unique. They all have their own likes and dislikes as far as food groups are concerned, and they all have different exercise levels and genetic backgrounds. That said, I do believe that every diet has some good features as well as some problems.

The Atkins Diet certainly is one of the most well known. Since Dr. Atkins[7] published his first book in 1972, there has been a tremendous controversy as to the role of dietary fat and carbohydrate. Dr. Atkins has often been dismissed as a renegade by the medical community. More recently there has been a renewed interest in his dietary theories. The Atkins Diet promotes a markedly restricted carbohydrate intake. The success of the Atkins Diet is in large part due to the restricted carbohydrate intake. Many people have been able to achieve weight loss with the Atkins Diet and I believe if you are able to achieve weight loss with this diet and have not had a significant rise in your serum cholesterol, it certainly is a reasonable program for you to follow.

There are however, several problems associated with the Atkins Diet. The first problem to consider is using the Atkins Diet in conjunction with athletic activities. The Atkins Diet, by its nature, causes the body to reduce its stored sugar levels. These stored sugars, in the form of glycogen, are often utilized while the body is exercising. Patients of mine who have used the Atkins Diet tended to have a significant drop in their energy level associated with exercise. It is, however, a reasonable diet for people who lead a sedentary lifestyle or have sedentary job activity.

The other major concern I have always had with the Atkins Diet is what exactly happens to a patient's cholesterol level. There are individual patients who follow this diet and because of their heavy consumption of fat can have a rise in cholesterol levels. For my particular patient population as a cardiologist, this is an adverse effect and the diet is not acceptable in that regard. There is one final observation that I would make on the Atkins Diet.

Although patients are able, at times, to lose a considerable amount of weight in spite of eating a high proportion of dietary fat, the basic concept of calories in – calories out, still applies. Patients taking in calories in the form of fat are taking in 9 calories per gram. If the same patients who are able to lose weight consuming one-half pound of bacon per day, changed their dietary intake to one-quarter pound of turkey, they would get nearly the same amount of protein but they would get dramatically less fat intake. That would promote faster weight loss and also a reduction in blood fat levels.

The Zone Diet is promoted by Dr. Barry Sears and I believe it is the most nutritionally balanced for the majority of my patients and probably for the majority of Americans. The Zone Diet promotes a calorie intake of 40-30-30. As you look at the spectrum of diets in Table 4, I propose that the majority of Americans would be able to achieve weight control following the recommended Zone ratios. Just like many other genetic attributes, I believe our ability to consume carbohydrates is probably a bell-shaped curve. I suspect the peak of the bell curve is between 40 and 50% carbohydrate intake with the smaller aspects of the bell stretching out to 70-80% carbohydrate on the right and possibly down to 20% carbohydrate on the left. That is to say that some patients are able to consume 70-80% carbohydrate without gaining any weight and some patients, even if they consume 30% carbohydrate will gain weight. Where you are on the bell-shaped curve is determined in part by your genetics and further manipulated by your exercise pattern.

I strongly recommend the Zone style diet for patients interested in athletic performance. I routinely recommend it to my friends who compete in athletics. I previously recommended the diet to my patients and still do on occasion. The major downfall of the Zone Diet for many of my patients is the necessity to measure food, weigh food and use a calculator. Although some patients ultimately need to resort to those techniques because of difficulty in achieving weight loss, I believe the majority of people who try an exercise and diet program are able to lose weight without having to do more than read labels on the food they eat. Ultimately, I derived the three principles covered in the next chapter, because of my patient's frustration in applying the principles of the Zone Diet.

Weight Watchers is an excellent program. I have a fondness in my heart for Weight Watchers because my mother was always able to achieve success through them. Anything that made mom happy, made the Gavin boys happy. My brothers and I actually grew up in part eating Weight Watchers approved menus. Weight Watchers is an excellent program for people who need a group support mechanism. It does, however, involve meetings and fees and many of my individual patients were not interested in following that kind of structured program. I should note that the majority of my patients are male, and Weight Watchers tends to be a female dominated organization. If Weight Watchers works for you, it is a great program.

The American Heart Association Diet is a diet that is

TABLE 5

The Food Pyramid

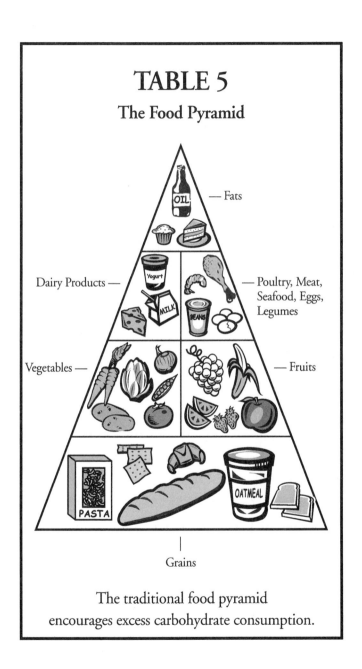

Fats

Dairy Products

Poultry, Meat, Seafood, Eggs, Legumes

Vegetables

Fruits

Grains

The traditional food pyramid
encourages excess carbohydrate consumption.

relatively high in carbohydrates and low in fat. But even though the diet is low in fat, it is high in energy, and those calories are very easily converted to fat within the body. The American Heart Association Diet and the food pyramid that is proposed by the USDA and noted in Table 5, both attain a relatively high percentage of their calories through carbohydrates. Some of my patients can tolerate a diet like that, however, the majority, in my opinion, seem to gain weight. A very simple question to ask yourself is, "Have you have been following the American Heart Association Diet and gaining weight?" If you have been gaining weight, then this is probably not the right diet for you.

I have also seen a very unfortunate diet approach develop that you should be aware of. Patients become frustrated with their inability to lose weight on the standard American Diabetic Association Diet or the American Heart Association Diet. These patients then jump all the way to the Atkins Diet and are often able to lose significant amounts of weight. Unfortunately, these patients then return to their former eating habits and regain the weight they lost. This cycle of weight gain and weight loss becomes relentless and demoralizing. These patients should move themselves long-term into a 40-30-30 style program and stay there.

As I noted earlier, there is no perfect diet. Each diet seems to have its strong points and also its weak points. I do think it is helpful to try to consider what type of diet you are eating now and what are the relative proportions of the various food groups. As people try to deal with weight loss, it seems to be helpful to lower your carbohydrate intake and move to the diets more to the left of where you are now. It also helps to increase your exercise level. If you are gaining weight and eating in a given range of carbohydrate percentage and are already doing an exercise program which is reasonable, then I believe it is even more important to cut down the carbohydrate intake in your diet.

Chapter Six
THE THREE RULE DIET

I developed the Three Rule Diet because my patients came back to my office frustrated that they did not understand the various diet books that I had recommended to them. I soon realized that patients did not want to use a calculator, weigh food, or buy special foods. As noted in the earlier chapter, there are a number of similarities between the various diets. I tried to distill down the various diets into their core principles and then have patients apply those principles to the foods they liked. Although you will not have to weigh or measure food on a regular basis with this diet, you will need to be aware of what you are eating.

It is important to recognize how much protein or carbohydrate you might be eating in a given meal, but the good news is you simply need to read. Because of government regulations, most of the foods you eat, with the exception of vegetables and fruits, come with the number of calories in a given serving of food and further categorize it with the number of calories that are contributed from carbohydrate, fat and protein. By simply looking at the box of cereal or the container of yogurt, you quickly will find out the calories and the breakdown of the foods you are eating.

The first rule is you must eat three meals a day. I know that seems very simple, but many of my patients skip breakfast or lunch and some patients in my practice formerly only ate one meal per day – dinner. The effect of eating a large number of calories at the end of your day has been studied in animals but not in humans. Rats that are fed three equal caloric meals throughout the day tend to have a normal body weight. Rats that are fed the same total calories as one large meal at the end of the day are fat.

The important point is that eating the majority of your calorie intake late in the day is associated with obesity. That occurs even if you are eating an appropriate amount of calories per day. A recent survey showed that skipping breakfast is a marker for obesity and diabetes. If you want to skip a meal, skip dinner. The simplest diet I know is actually to not eat after 4:00 in the afternoon. I have known people to adopt this principle and have successful weight loss over the long term. It is a very difficult style of eating to follow for various social and physical reasons.

I stress the importance of breakfast and lunch, because people who skip breakfast or lunch tend to overeat at night. These people literally starve themselves through the day, and then when they get home begin consuming large amounts of food. I have one patient who only ate one meal a day, dinner, and now eats two meals a day. She eats breakfast and lunch, and is no longer hungry enough to eat dinner. She has lost considerable weight. For people who have a difficult time eating breakfast, either because of habit or time constraints, I recommend they try eating peanut butter on a piece of toast. Peanut butter on toast is an excellent breakfast option. The combination of peanut butter and toast gives a relatively balanced meal between carbohydrate, protein and fat. It is also quick and easy to make for people on the go. By eating breakfast you fire up your metabolic engine and make it easier for your body to burn excess fat.

Rule number two is eat some lean protein with every meal. This is often one of the more difficult rules for patients to adopt. The challenge is for you to define what type of lean protein you like. The protein source can be meat, fish, fowl or even peanut butter. If it is a vegetable source such as peanut butter or soy nut butter, you need to insure that it has at least 7-8 grams of protein per serving. There are all types of lean protein sources available, but what is very important is that it has to be a protein source that you like. Examples of lean protein might include egg whites, peanut butter, smoked fish, Canadian bacon, lean lunch meat, nonfat yogurt, low-fat cottage cheese, mozzarella cheese, not to mention multiple types of meat, fish or fowl.

I stress to my patients the need to eat lean protein because it will keep you from getting hungry until the next meal. I ask my patients to do a simple experiment. One morning, have two pieces of toast or a bagel for breakfast. Write down on a piece of paper how many hours after breakfast you get hungry. The next morning, have one piece of toast or one-half bagel for breakfast but put peanut butter on it. You will find that you will not get hungry for an additional two hours. I have experienced this effect personally.

When I was heavy, I used to eat a bagel for breakfast at roughly 6:00 in the morning. I often would get to the hospital and start work by 7:00 and often by 8:30-9:00 I would be hungry. As I was walking through the doctors' lounge at 8:30 or 9:00, I would often walk by a plate of donuts and pastries and pick one up. I was, after all, hungry. Now that I eat lean protein with my breakfast every morning, I walk by the same plate of donuts and I have no interest in them. By eating the lean protein with your meal, you will not be hungry for an additional 2-3 hours. What I have found personally is, it is very easy not to eat if you are not hungry. I would also point out that the converse of that statement is true. It is very difficult to continue to avoid food when you are hungry and food choices people make for snacking are often poor. I believe a major problem of the diets that are high in carbohydrate and low in protein is they cause people to be excessively hungry between meals.

Rule three is no white at night. Patients often look at me a little confused after I tell them this rule. I want you to think about what is white. No white at night means no rice, bread, potatoes or pasta. It also applies to all the colored variants of those foods. Also banned at your evening meal would be red potatoes, brown rice, whole wheat bread and the starchy vegetables such as corn, which I might note comes in a white variety! Dinner should become lean

41

meat, fish, or fowl and all the salad and vegetables you want.

You might be thinking, "Why do we need to limit starch intake?" Starch is, after all, a low-fat food group. When we send cattle to Nebraska to fatten them up, what do we feed them? The stockyards feed those animals low-fat grain. Those cattle are mammals just like us. The cattle producers do not feed the animals lard, nor do they feed them vegetable oil. Yet, those same animals dramatically increase their fat content. In Lewis County, south of my hometown, the local hog producers feed their hogs old bread purchased from the Safeway stores. There is *NO* fat in a loaf of bread. Yet again, the hogs also mammals, add to their body fat by eating the bread.

The explanation for the conversion process of sugar to fat is efficiency. Our bodies do not store significant amounts of energy in sugar. The body does have some sugar stores, called glycogen, which are located in the liver to supply the brain sugar in times of emergency, and also in the muscles to be burned if the flight or fight system is activated. The majority of our energy stores are in body fat.

In a kilogram (2.2 pounds) of glycogen there are 5,000 calories. In a kilogram of body fat there are 9,000 calories. In the same weight, the body is able to carry nearly twice the stored energy in fat than it can in sugar. A significant reason for this is because fat is relatively dehydrated. The stored glycogen has water with it so it can be burned immediately in times of emergency.

I ask patients to think of the concept of a thousand pennies. If I were to give you a thousand pennies, how would you carry those pennies around? I would suspect that by the end of the day, those pennies would be converted into ten paper bills. That would be a much more efficient way for you to carry that money. Your body is basically doing the same thing. Your body converts any excess sugar calories to fat within twenty-four hours.

A concept that should not be forgotten here is that you can get fat eating no-fat foods. No different than the hogs or the cattle, humans can gain weight and store body fat if fed a diet that is high in carbohydrates. As you walk through a supermarket, you will be inundated with bright, colorful labels touting low-fat or reduced-fat foods. No-fat foods can still be loaded with energy in the form of carbohydrates. Although that food source may go through your mouth as no fat, your body will not store it that way.

All food sources are broken down into a universal energy and then ideally stored as body fat if the body has excess calories. It is relatively straightforward and easy for the body to store the energy of carbohydrates or fat that is taken orally. It is more difficult for the body to store protein calories as body fat. The process to break down protein to a simple energy source has a significant energy consumption and the net return in storing protein calories as fat is not very efficient for the body. Do not, however, make the assumption that eating protein will build your muscles. Eating protein will allow you to have additional calories that you can burn for energy. To build your muscles you will have to engage in an exercise program and consume protein at the same time.

Another important point is the need to drink large amounts of water. The human body needs to have at least one liter of water per day for minimal existence. Most nutritional programs recommend that you drink eight large glasses of water per day. This is certainly reasonable. Remember, your body is predominantly water. If you are trying to burn body fat, you need to drink even more water.

As noted above, a kilogram of body fat contains 9,000 calories. If you were in a starvation mode, you could live for nine days on that amount of calories. To adequately burn that fat requires adding at least a liter of water per day. Thus, to burn 2.2 pounds of fat, you need to consume nearly twenty pounds of water. Stored body fat is an extremely efficient light energy source that can be unlocked with adequate amounts of water.

A good rule is to try to balance the calories between your three meals throughout the day. If your diet is going to consist of 1800 calories, have roughly 400-500 calories at every meal. Depending on what time you eat dinner, you may note that you begin to get hungry at 4:00-5:00. If you know that your dinner is going to be late, try to have some type of snack that has a significant protein content between 4:00 and 5:00 in the afternoon. In chapter 9, we will give you some very practical examples of what sorts of food you can eat at various meals. If you were going to slant your calorie intake towards one part of the day or another, I would encourage you to slant your largest meal to be breakfast and your smallest meal to be dinner.

There is an old saying among people who counsel dieters, "Eat breakfast like a king, lunch like a storekeeper and dinner like a pauper." By putting the majority of your calories early in the day, you have the greatest opportunity to burn them off. By delaying your calorie intake to the latter part of the day, you give your body the greatest opportunity to store the extra calories. If you make the evening meal high in starches such as rice, bread or pasta, you further drive the hormonal mechanisms of the body to store those calories as fat.

By reducing the starch in your diet you will change the glycemic index of the foods you are eating. The glycemic index of food groups is probably important to all people trying to lose weight, and especially to diabetic patients. The glycemic index of a given food group is a measurement of how fast your blood sugar rises after you eat that food group. The faster your blood sugar rises, the higher the glycemic index of that particular food.[8] The food with the highest glycemic index would be sugar in water. Potatoes, white bread and rice have a very high glycemic index. Foods with a high glycemic index produce a very high insulin response within your body. That insulin rise leads ultimately to hypoglycemia and hunger several hours later. In addition, insulin is the primary hormone in driving production of body fat from excess calories. Changing the carbohydrates in your diet at night from starch such as rice, bread or potatoes to vegetables or salad, reduces your insulin level and may help promote weight loss.

Another important concept to understand in conjunction with the glycemic index, is glycemic load. Glycemic load is the measurement of the total carbohydrate or sugar in a given food group. Food groups may have a high glycemic index but a low amount of total carbohydrate or glycemic load. For example, potatoes have a high glycemic index and also have a high glycemic load. Thus, the rise in your blood sugar after eating a meal with potatoes will be relatively high and sustained. Carrots have a high glycemic index, nearly as high as that of potatoes. Carrots, however, have a low glycemic load. The potential spike that can be produced in your blood sugar from eating a certain amount of carrots may be sharp, but it will not be particularly prolonged. That is why some people consider carrots *bad* in your diet when trying to lose weight. In reality, the glycemic load of carrots is so low, they are not a particular problem. You will not get fat eating carrots.

In the public press you will often see the glycemic index of various food groups. Unfortunately, you will not often see the glycemic load of those same food groups. I do believe eating a low glycemic index diet will help you lose weight. Eating low glycemic index foods will decrease your insulin levels and that should make it easier for you to lose weight. There have been multiple books written about the concept of glycemic index and how it can effect weight loss. A good research tool for learning more about the glycemic index and glycemic load of various food groups is the Internet. If you search the Internet under glycemic index you will find several sites that list hundreds of food groups. I would especially urge you, if you are a diabetic patient, to learn more about low glycemic index foods and favor them in your diet.

In my own diet, I have definitely moved to lower glycemic index foods. I eat less starch such as bagels or pastries in the morning. I also rarely eat rice, bread or potatoes any more at night. Instead of eating starch at night I eat carbohydrate in the form of vegetables or salad. In reality, I have reduced not only my glycemic index but also my glycemic load. Although I cannot *prove* that this has made a difference in my weight, I will note that my body fat is the lowest it has been in twenty years and I believe it has made a significant difference in my ability to lose weight and ability to maintain my present weight. Ironically, I used to believe that the problem with the baked potato was the extras like butter or sour cream that you put on it. Now I believe the potato is just as big of a problem as the extras.

Patients also ask me how much lean protein is enough. I ask patients to eat *reasonable* quantities of lean protein. A rule of thumb might be to eat a number of grams of protein as high as one-half your weight in pounds. If you are very athletic you may need to increase your protein intake to one gram of protein per pound. You certainly do not need to consume more protein than that. Most patients I see are not consuming excess protein. By stressing the need to eat lean protein at every meal including breakfast, my average patient probably increases his or her overall protein intake. At your evening meal, a chicken breast or 4-6 ounces of fish or meat is more than adequate. I find it ironic now that when I go out to a restaurant that specializes in steak, I usually am ordering the "petite fillet" which is often 8 ounces and not uncommonly the smallest steak on the menu.

Fruits are high in fiber and vitamins and are a good supplement to any diet. I would, however, ask you to restrict drinking of fruit juices. I would avoid orange juice because it is high in sugar. I would also avoid fruits that are high in sugar and release their sugar very fast into the blood stream. These fruits have a high glycemic index. These fruits might include, grapes, raisins, oranges, peaches, nectarines, and tangerines. Pears and apples should be favored as they have a lower glycemic index. The sugar will be released slower into the blood stream due to the fiber content.

I encourage patients to restrict their starch intake to the equivalent of one slice of bread at breakfast and lunch. That starch can be in any number of forms, such as an English muffin, half a bagel, or a bowl of oatmeal. I would encourage you to favor breads or cereals that are not refined. I would favor whole grain products, stone ground products, oatmeal and avoid products based on white flour. By doing this you will increase the fiber content in your diet and you will reduce the initial sugar load that your body experiences after a meal. By changing diet in this way, many patients, myself included, have found that they no longer become sleepy after a meal. My energy level is relatively constant for 4-5 hours and I no longer get hungry 2-3 hours after eating.

I have asked you with these *three rules* to limit the amount of starch in your diet. I have also limited the amount of fat in your diet by asking you to eat lean protein sources. I will not restrict the amount of vegetables or salad in your diet. You can eat unlimited amounts of nonstarchy vegetables and unlimited amounts of salad with this diet. There are carbohydrates or sugars in vegetables but it is so interwoven with fiber that it is released relatively slowly and the amount of sugar is not that great. Granted, there is more sugar in carrots than celery, but I have never known anyone who has gotten fat eating carrots. So, regardless of the meal, you can eat as much salad or vegetables as you choose.

Patients often ask about the use of salad dressing. This clearly is a source of dietary fat intake. I would encourage you to find a low-fat or even nonfat salad dressing that you like. Try to use salad dressings that have a significant amount of vinegar content. I would note that if your major fat intake at night is in the form of salad dressing, you will have markedly restricted your fat intake.

I would also note that the same hormone system involved in breaking down your body's fat which is mediated by a hormone called glucagon is also responsible for breaking down the dietary fat that you are eating at night. There is significant controversy in the medical literature about what is the right amount of fat for people to consume. It may be that consuming a small but reasonable amount of fat is helpful in keeping your fat burning system activated and primed.

Patients often ask me if it is allowable to drink alcoholic beverages such as wine or hard liquor on this diet. It is important to note that alcoholic beverages have a significant carbohydrate load. All the calories in alcoholic beverages are in the form of carbohydrates. Two glasses of wine is fundamentally equal to a large baked potato. For the purpose of weight loss, complete abstinence from alcohol is probably ideal. If you do choose to drink a limited amount of alcohol while actively dieting, then you will need to either increase your exercise or acknowledge that your weight loss may be slower over time.

I actually encourage many of my patients with cardiovascular disease to drink ½ glass of red wine in the evening. When I was actively trying to lose weight, that was the amount of wine that I would consume. Once you have achieved your weight loss target, you can then consider increasing your starch intake or increase your alcohol intake. A very reasonable approach is to consume your carbohydrate as an alcoholic beverage at dinnertime. That may be 1-2 mixed drinks or 1-2 glasses of wine. In the past, there was a relatively popular diet referred to as the drinking man's diet which promoted carbohydrate restriction other than alcohol in the evening.

Patients also ask me if they need to utilize a multivitamin. The majority of patients following these dietary principles will actually increase their vegetable intake. It certainly is reasonable to consider consuming a once-a-day adult multiple vitamin. I would also propose that you consider reviewing your common foodstuffs during the day. If you eat a diet that is relatively low in milk or dairy products, you may also want to consider using a calcium supplement. Other than an adult multivitamin and calcium supplementation, it is unlikely that the majority of patients will need additional vitamins. If you believe in using additional vitamin supplements, that is acceptable. The added vitamins will probably not harm you and you can decide the benefit versus cost.

More important than vitamins is how dieting may effect your medications. The foods favored by the diet should not effect your medications, but your weight loss will. Your need for medication for high blood pressure, diabetes, and high cholesterol may decrease dramatically with weight loss. As your weight drops check your blood pressure more frequently, and check with your doctor about decreasing your medications. If you have diabetes be sure to read the chapter on diabetic patients. Dealing with the need to decrease your medications is a good problem to have.

A common problem for some of my patients is trying to figure out how their daily work schedule meshes with these dietary principles. For those patients who have irregular sleep hours such as long haul truck drivers or those who work graveyard shift, I would propose the following consideration. After awakening from what is your normal sleep time, consider your first meal to be your breakfast meal. It is quite appropriate to consume some starch with that meal. You still need to follow the other principles and also consume some lean protein at that meal. At the last meal of your work shift, consume no starch. You should consider that meal to be your supper meal. That meal should consist of some lean protein and again, all the salad or vegetables you choose.

In summary then, I recommend that you follow three simple principles in your eating: eat three meals per day, consume a reasonable portion of lean protein with every meal, and finally, eat no white (starch) at night. Try to consume no more than the equivalent of one slice of bread at breakfast and lunch. Eat all the salad and non-starchy vegetables that you choose. Finally, increase your consumption of water and fruits. If you apply these principles to foods that you like, you should find the changes in your diet relatively simple. I developed these rules to help people achieve weight loss in a simple way, and I am happy to say that when patients return and have lost weight, they commonly tell me, "it's not that hard." I believe you can do it too.

When a patient comes to my office I give them my instructions for exercise and the three rules of the diet written on a prescription blank. I do that to emphasize to the patients that I believe their diet and exercise pattern is as important as any medication I may prescribe. I ask those people to put that prescription on their refrigerator door. At the back of this book on page 91 you will find your *prescription*. Place it on your refrigerator door, and follow it.

Chapter Seven
LONG TERM WEIGHT CONTROL

The success of any diet or weight loss program should not be measured in short-term weight loss, but long-term weight control. You may be able to reach your target weight loss over the next 3-6 months by following the *three rule* diet, but what is most important to me is that you are able to keep your weight off over time. Many patients will lose a considerable amount of weight only to slowly gain it back over time.

As I noted earlier, your current body weight is a reflection of your long-term calorie intake and calorie expenditure. Patients are able to achieve significant weight loss by increasing their calorie expenditure over a long period of time and bringing down their own body fat stores. What is important in the weight loss process is recognizing what has been the key to your success. For patients who achieve weight loss by markedly restricting their calorie intake and using a calorie source such as a liquid diet supplement, which deviates from their normal eating and social pattern, it is very likely they are going to regain their weight when they return to their old patterns. The more your weight loss program deviates from what you would normally eat, the more likely you are to regain your weight. I personally do not perceive myself to be on a diet anymore, but I did significantly change the way I ate several years ago.

Fortunately, for most patients, the weight loss process will take a significant amount of time. In my own case, I lost ten pounds over one year, and then lost roughly thirty-five pounds over the next fourteen months. The entire time was in excess of two years. During that time I discovered foods that I enjoyed eating and a way of eating that kept my energy level high, met my caloric needs, and did not involve getting hungry between meals. I would hope that the same process would happen to you.

A realistic expectation is that someone can lose between thirty and fifty pounds over the course of a year. As noted earlier, body fat has a very high energy content. If you expend an extra 325 calories per day, you will lose on the order of twenty-five pounds over the course of a year. You need to lose in excess of 650 calories per day to lose fifty pounds per year. Weight loss in excess of fifty pounds per year is very difficult to achieve, except for patients who are extremely obese. Patients commonly weighing greater than 350 pounds actually have significant amounts of muscle mass needed to support their large body structures. When these patients lose weight, they not only lose body fat but they also lose muscle mass. Muscle mass, because of its higher water content, gives greater weight loss. I tell patients if they can achieve a weight loss of 2-4 pounds per month, they are doing quite well.

After you have achieved a weight goal that you are happy with, you can begin to modify your diet. A core principle to the diet during the period of weight loss is *no white at night.* When you have reached your target weight, you can begin to re-introduce a limited portion of starch into your supper or evening meal. That may be a small portion of potatoes or rice, or it may be an increased amount of alcohol. Remember, two bottles of beer has the same calorie equivalent as a baked potato. Whatever starch group you choose to add, add only one and add it in a reasonable portion. Then monitor your weight over the next several weeks and months. If you are consuming the right amount of calories, your weight will level off and you should be back to a steady state. If your weight begins to rise, then you have added too much starch and you will need to move your eating habits back to those closer aligned with what you were following when you were losing weight.

The good news is that during your period of weight loss, you will probably discover some foods you like and find you do not miss those high-energy starches as you thought you would. In my case, I discovered that adding protein to my breakfast kept me from getting hungry until noon. I also learned about yogurt and string cheese from a friend; it is now my standard lunch. By the time you need to deal with the weight maintenance versus weight loss, you will be eating in a different way and should have discovered foods that you like and eating patterns that work for you. If you return to your former exercise pattern and also your former eating pattern, you will undoubtedly return to your former weight.

Just as it took several months or even years for you to lose the weight, it will take months and years for you to put the weight back on, but it will return. In losing weight you will have discovered what types of foods you can eat and control your weight, but you will not have changed your underlying genetic structure. That will remain with you for life. But you will have the knowledge and power to control your weight if you choose to. In the later chapter, So What Should I Eat?, I will show you some examples of how I changed my eating at various meals and then how I changed my food intake when I reached my target weight.

Chapter Eight
THE DIABETIC PATIENT

Diabetic patients have some unique medical issues involving diet and weight. I have a special empathy for my diabetic patients. My mother is a diabetic. I also have a family history of adult onset diabetes. Unfortunately, the incidence of diabetes and obesity is going up across the country and many patients seem to have a poor understanding of their illness.

Diabetes is a weight driven illness. In a recent issue of the *Journal of the American Medical Association*[9], a survey study showed that the number of American adults who are obese continues to rise across the country. Not surprisingly, the number of US adults who are diabetic continues to increase in both sexes, all ages, and all races. It is important to understand that diabetes is not a uniform illness. If any of you have ever known a diabetic child, that is an individual who had diabetes occur in grade school or high school more than five years ago, I will make a uniform prediction that that individual was thin.

Children with diabetes have a lack of insulin due to some type of autoimmune process where they destroy their own pancreas. These children cannot make insulin to help control their blood sugar level. Also they cannot make insulin to help promote storage of body fat. Typically when these children are diagnosed with new onset diabetes, they are thin and have just lost a considerable amount of weight.

Adults who are diagnosed with diabetes have a much greater diversity in their illness. The majority of these adults are overweight. These adults tend to have normal or even high insulin levels but they have lost sensitivity to the insulin levels in their end organ tissues or they simply cannot make enough insulin for the size of their bodies. Insulin's role in the body is not only to control blood sugar but also to control body fat. The more body fat one has, the higher the level of insulin required to manage it. The most straightforward way to help a diabetic patient who is overweight is to help them lose weight. By losing weight the patient can then bring their body size into better balance with the level of insulin that his or her own pancreas can produce.

Patients that I meet with diabetes often are considerably overweight. Commonly they are 20-30% over their ideal body weight, having at least an extra 40-60 pounds of body fat. These individuals often are referred to me because they have had poor control of their hypertension. Not surprisingly, these patients have all the illnesses attributed to obesity. They commonly have hypertension as well as high cholesterol and possibly underlying cardiovascular disease. When I first talk to these patients I commonly ask them if anyone has ever told them that they should lose weight. The common answer is actually, "yes."

I then ask them if anyone has ever told them how to lose weight and the response to that is typically, "no." I then ask them two other questions that I think are very important. I ask them if anyone has ever explained to them that if they lose 40-60 pounds, their diabetes could go away. The typical response to that answer is "no." Finally, I ask the diabetic patient if he or she was ever on a diabetic diet and gained weight on that diet. The common response is "yes."

In Chapter five we reviewed the various diets touted to the American public. The diet proposed to most patients by the American Diabetic Association is relatively high in carbohydrate and starch. That diet, in essence, was designed for children who were thin and had relatively insignificant insulin levels. Most adults with adult onset diabetes are obese and some of them even have high insulin levels. I believe the majority of Americans would actually gain weight on the American Diabetic Association diet. I know I would, and I have seen many patients gain weight on this diet.

If you are a diabetic patient following the standard diabetic diet, you are consuming a large amount of your calories as starch and carbohydrate. If you have been gaining weight on this diet, or had difficulty in losing weight on this diet, you need to move your diet to the left side of Table 4 in the diet spectrum. By reducing your starch and carbohydrate intake you will probably find it easier to control your blood sugars and you will also find it easier to lose weight. As I stated in the prior chapter, it is very important to adopt a diet with lower glycemic index foods if you are diabetic. That will decrease your need for insulin and help you lose weight.

For those patients who simply have high blood sugar and have been counseled by their doctor to lose weight, you can follow my diet principles and that should be adequate. For those diabetic patients who are currently on medication you will need to work with your doctor towards reducing your medication. If you are a diabetic patient and 40-60 pounds overweight and only taking oral medication, there is the potential that you can get rid of your need for medication by losing weight.

What many patients do not understand is that by being on the diabetic medication and eating a high carbohydrate diet, they are actually more inclined to gain weight than to lose weight. Think back to when you initially were diagnosed with diabetes. If you gained weight after your doctor started new medication, then you were eating too much carbohydrate in your diet for your own personal metabolism. In addition, the medicines can also make people hungry by raising your insulin level. Unfortunately patients get trapped into a progressive tailspin. They get put on more medication, they get hungrier, they eat more, and they gain more weight. As they gain weight, their blood sugars go up and then they get put on more medication. It is a relentless cycle.

To break the cycle, you need to change your diet. By changing your diet, reducing your carbohydrate/starch intake, you will first notice that your blood sugars come under better control. If you work with your doctor to try and reduce your medications, you will then find that it will be easier to lose weight. The ultimate goal for any obese diabetic patient should be to try and manage blood sugars with no medication at all. To do that you will have to lose weight. By taking oral medication for control of blood sugar, the diabetic patient does reduce the risk of kidney and eye disease. Unfortunately the leading cause of death among diabetic patients is cardiovascular disease and simply controlling the blood sugar with oral agents or insulin does not decrease the diabetic patient's risk of cardiovascular disease.

I have actually had overweight patients who were counseled to eat more when their blood sugar levels dropped to very low levels. It is somewhat of a chicken and an egg concept. Which should happen first? Should the doctor lower the patient's medication or should the patient try to follow a better diet? If your blood sugar levels are high, you will need to follow a better diet before your doctor will be able to lower your medication dosages. If your blood sugar levels are already well maintained and you are eating a diet relatively high in starch and you are overweight, ask your doctor about starting a better diet and simultaneously cutting back some of your medication.

One of my own success stories is a patient who was significantly overweight, taking 100 units of insulin twice a day, with relatively poor blood sugar control. After explaining the concepts of his illness to him and working with his diet, he ultimately lost sixty-five pounds and now uses 30 units or less of insulin twice daily. His blood sugar levels are near normal. I am not sure if this individual patient will be able to completely escape the use of medication or insulin, but his insulin therapy is markedly lowered and his blood sugar levels are much better controlled.

I ask my diabetic patients to follow my three basic rules. I do believe that the diabetic diet has too much starch or carbohydrate in it for patients who are gaining weight on that diet. There is one positive aspect of the diabetic diet — it teaches you the concept of carbohydrate substitution. I ask my diabetic patients to eat no more than one slice of bread or its equivalent with breakfast and lunch. The rule of no white at night still applies, and diabetics can consume all the salad and non-starchy vegetables they choose at night. It is especially important for diabetics to avoid sugary fruits that raise blood sugar levels quickly such as oranges, grapes, and raisins. Patients with diabetes should especially strive to follow a diet that favors low glycemic index foods. Those foods will cause fewer glucose spikes and should require less insulin to maintain normal blood sugars.

An exercise program is important for anyone who wants to lose weight. An exercise program is especially important for diabetic patients. Exercise helps drive blood sugar levels down by driving the blood sugar into the muscle groups. Developing an exercise program such as walking will help lower your blood sugar levels and help decrease your need for insulin or medication. Combining an exercise program with a change in your diet will only speed the process of losing weight.

Diabetes is an illness often caused by obesity in adults. If you can treat your obesity, you can often markedly improve or possibly even eradicate your diabetes. Losing weight is more difficult for diabetic patients if they are on medication. Weight loss becomes a balancing act between exercise, diet and a gradual reduction in your diabetes medication. The most important person in that balancing act is you, the patient. By changing your exercise pattern and diet you will have better control of your blood sugar and make it easier for your physician to lower your diabetes medicine. You will probably find it relatively slow-going at first but as your diabetes medicine levels go down, your weight loss will get easier. Almost uniformly when patients stop their diabetes medications and are following a good diet and exercise program, their weight loss will accelerate.

Chapter Nine
SO DOC, WHAT SHOULD I EAT?

Now that you've heard the three rules to the diet, you should start to think about how you are going to apply them to yourself. As I stated earlier in the book, this is about finding foods that you like and that meet the criteria of the three rules. As you go through this chapter, write down what you eat now at each meal and analyze it. Does what you eat now fit with the three rules? If not, think about how you can modify what you are eating. As you read this chapter, write down some reasonable options for you to eat at every meal.

You will need to learn more about what you are eating. With the nutrition facts printed on most food packages, it is not difficult to understand the breakdown of that food group. I would like to review some basics of food label reading with you. The label will tell you the *total* number of calories. It will also tell you the components of the food such as fat, carbohydrate and protein. Unfortunately the components are not given as a percentage of total calories so you cannot readily apply the concept of the 40-30-30 balance without doing some simple math. The absolute amounts of protein, fat or carbohydrate are given by weight in grams and that is useful. If you intend to use a given food group as a protein source, make sure that it has adequate protein. Any meal should have a minimum of 10-20 grams of protein.

It is important to remember that you will be combining some foods to make a meal. Let's use the example of nonfat yogurt and string cheese. The yogurt is 110 calories with no fat. The yogurt has 20 grams of carbohydrate and 7 grams of protein per serving. The string cheese has 80 calories per tube and contains 6 grams of fat and 7 grams of protein per serving. The combination of yogurt and two tubes of string cheese is an overall excellent meal and reasonably balanced. The combination produces 20 grams of carbohydrate, 21 grams of protein, and 12 grams of fat.

I arrived at this combination with some experimentation over time and did not really check the exact content of the food groups until after I had been eating this for lunch for at least six months. Although the exact percentages are not 40-30-30, they are close enough. The 40-30-30 percentages are a good target, but we can certainly vary that meal to meal. Use the nutritional facts in labels to give you some general guidelines. Then, check the numbers more closely on specific food groups that you really like. If you are doing well with your weight loss program, don't sweat the small stuff. If you are struggling with your weight loss, you need to pay attention to the details.

I would propose some general guidelines that you can consider when you look at the absolute number of grams of the various food groups. Remember that you are trying to target a 40-30-30 balance. It does *not* have to be exact.

The important point is whether this meal satisfies your hunger and keeps you from getting hungry for an additional four to five hours. Add up the various categories of carbohydrate, protein and fat from the various food serving groups that you are eating. A good rule of thumb is that at least every meal should have at least 10-20 grams of carbohydrate. The amount of protein in grams should be slightly higher but no lower than three-fourths the amount of carbohydrate. Remember, protein has only 4 calories per gram versus 5 calories for carbohydrate. Finally, the amount of fat should be roughly one-half of the amount of carbohydrate. These simple proportions will allow you to come close to the 40-30-30 rules for any given snack or meal.

Usually the hardest part of the diet is finding the lean protein sources you like, so let's start with breakfast. People usually have some type of starch they eat with breakfast. It may be toast, an English muffin, or oatmeal. I would favor the oatmeal or some type of non-white, whole grain bread. Good breakfast protein sources are Canadian bacon, egg whites, peanut butter, soy nut butter if you are allergic to peanut butter, lox or turkey bacon. An excellent simple breakfast choice is peanut butter on a piece of whole wheat toast. Many of my patients do not eat breakfast. For those *breakfast impaired* individuals, I advise peanut butter on a piece of non-white toast. It is simple, and it is very balanced so you will not get hungry until lunch time.

If you are time constrained in the morning, try peanut butter on an English muffin. If you choose some type of processed meat like ground turkey sausage, be sure that it has low fat content. Simply look at the package and check the component percentages. Remember I said you would not have to use a calculator, but you will have to read labels.

I would like to make some special points about eggs. Eggs are often maligned in the public press. Egg whites are a wonderful balanced source of protein. You can literally live on egg whites as your only source of protein. They are also a relatively inexpensive source of protein. An egg yolk is a 200 mg cholesterol pill. All the protein in the egg is in the whites and all the cholesterol is in the yolk. If you like eggs, consider having three in the morning but only one yolk per day. If you have a medical condition that mandates a very reduced cholesterol intake, try the egg whites alone. For those who do not want to hassle separating eggs, consider Egg Beaters.

Personally, I eat three hard-boiled egg whites per day during the week. I make egg white omelets on the weekend when I have more time. You can really make the omelets flavorful with salsa, green onions or vegetables. If you want to add some cheese, try mozzarella. You can also add lean meat like Canadian bacon. I used to give our dog all the egg yolks until a veterinarian friend told me I would kill the dog, and now he only gets one. The dogs use the cholesterol for making the oils in their coat and they love the taste but remember, the limit is one per day.

You should try to get at least 10-20 grams of protein at your breakfast meal. Your breakfast protein will help keep you form being hungry until lunchtime. The worst breakfast choice that you could make is not to eat breakfast at all. By skipping a meal you are only increasing your likelihood of overeating later. You need to eat breakfast even if you are not hungry. If you have a significant time constraint in the morning, consider again a piece of toast with peanut butter or on an English muffin. It is quick and easy. If even that is too much of a time delay, consider using something like Carnation Instant Breakfast, Slim Fast, or some type of balanced breakfast bar that has a balance between the food groups of carbohydrate, protein and fat in the range of 40-30-30. Breakfast is your most important meal. Do not skip it, even if you are not hungry.

Lunch is a little more straightforward. Most people already know what type of protein sources they like. Excellent protein sources can include lean lunchmeat, tuna fish, low-fat cottage cheese, nonfat yogurt and string cheese. As I said before, this is not about what I like; this is about what you like. For those people who eat sandwiches, think about using just one slice of bread. Use the same amount of protein or meat but just have half a sandwich. Another option is to toast the bread and build your sandwich with the outer leaves of a head of lettuce providing the upper layer.

An excellent lunch for people on the run is nonfat yogurt and string cheese. I realize not all people like yogurt, but for those who do, I would strongly recommend that you try this. When you buy yogurt, make sure you read how much protein your favorite brand has. A co-worker in my office pointed out the wide variance in protein content between the different types of nonfat yogurt.

There was a marked range in the level of carbohydrate and protein for the same number of calories. I would strongly recommend that you find a nonfat yogurt that has on the order of 8-10 grams of protein per unit. If you add the string cheese to the nonfat yogurt it does add protein and fat to it, which gives a very good blend of carbohydrate, protein and fat. Personally, I favor nonfat yogurt and string cheese for lunch. I have found that by eating this I am usually not hungry for 4-5 hours and my energy level is excellent. I strongly recommend this lunch combination to people who are on the go or for my patients who are on the road, such as truck drivers. If you plan ahead, you will not have to make bad choices in foods available at fast food restaurants or convenience stores. Never skip lunch, even if you are not hungry. Skipping lunch, like skipping breakfast, just causes you to overeat later in the day.

Many times people get hungry at 4-5 o'clock and need a snack. I would strongly recommend that you consider eating some type of snack if your dinner is going to be delayed until 6-7 o'clock. By eating a balanced food between 4 and 5 o'clock, you will not get so hungry that you will make a bad food choice at 6:30-7:00 o'clock. I keep a box of Balance bars that are designed along the 40-40-30 blend in my office for those times when I know I am going to be late getting home. Other good snack alternatives can include cut up vegetables such as carrots or celery, celery and peanut butter, string cheese, peanuts or fruit such as bananas, pears, or apples. Bad choices for snacking would be something that is sugar based such as cookies, candy or carbonated soft drinks with sugar.

Remember to drink large amounts of water throughout the day. If you have had a previous habit of drinking numerous cans of a regular carbonated soft drink such as Coca-Cola or Pepsi throughout the day, stop it. The bad news is that those cans of soft drink each have 240 calories of sugar. The good news is that if you have been drinking that many cans of soda through the day, just stopping that alone will make a huge difference in your ability to lose weight. I have had friends or patients who have consumed at least a six-pack of a soft drink through the day. Those persons usually will lose a large amount of weight, on the order of twenty pounds in two months, as their sugar intake dramatically falls.

I personally favor any type of water-based drink including water with lemon or lime, iced tea, Crystal Lite, or any of the sugar-free soft drinks. There have been people in the medical literature that have theorized that the diet colas such as Diet Coke, Diet Pepsi, Diet RC, have some insulin-like properties. I previously used to consume Diet Coke or Pepsi at lunch and subsequently changed after reading those reports. I think if you want to optimize your chances of weight loss you should consider doing the same. Good choices are water or any of the non-cola diet soft drinks.

Dinner is probably the easiest meal for many people to apply the principles. You can have a reasonable portion of whatever lean protein source you like. It may be meat, fish or fowl. Common visual references would be fowl the size of a standard chicken breast. You could also consider pieces of meat the size of the palm of your hand or at least the size of a package of cigarettes. Being a cardiologist, I would strongly recommend that you think in terms of the size of the palm of your hand. Cooking techniques such as broiling or barbecuing are best, and a number of my patients use the cooking style espoused by the George Foreman Grill that drains away the fat as you cook.

Remember, you can have all the salad and non-starchy vegetables you want. Experiment with different salad dressings and different types of vinegar to find combinations you like. Try to use the lowest fat content salad dressings that taste good to you and use them in moderation. As I said before, this is about finding foods you like and can enjoy eating over the long term. It may take some time but I am sure you will be fascinated with how you come to appreciate foods that you had not thought about before.

You should forget about dessert. Personally, I have never understood why we would serve something that is high in sugar so late in the day and still do not eat dessert on any kind of regular basis. There may be special occasions when you are visiting a friend's house and they have prepared some special pie or cake. Consider taking a slice of the dessert home and having it for breakfast the next morning. Personally, I love apple pie and whenever some-one makes one and serves it at a dinner I am attending, I ask if I can bring home a slice for breakfast the next day. I do not eat it as dessert. In place of dessert consider having some fruit such as an apple or pear. Also, consider having a small piece of low-fat cheese.

I would like to make a special point about alcohol. Alcohol has a significant number of calories. The calories are entirely carbohydrate in nature. A glass of wine or a bottle of beer can easily be 180-240 calories. There are some beneficial changes in cholesterol levels associated with drinking one-half glass of red wine per day. For those people who are interested in optimizing their cholesterol status and choose to drink wine, I would suggest that you drink one-half glass of red wine after dinner.

Alcohol calories are relatively empty and they do not curb your hunger. By drinking your wine after dinner, you are more likely to enjoy it slowly and feel comfortable lim-iting yourself to only one-half glass. For those people who have been able to achieve an adequate degree of weight loss and are ready to start adding carbohydrate back into their evening meal, you can consider adding your carbo-hydrate as alcohol. A glass or two of wine or 1-2 bottles of beer are equivalent in calories to a baked potato. When I was a child the principle of drinking your carbohydrate calories was espoused in the popular Drinking Man's Diet.

Table 6 shows the foods I ate before I changed my diet, as well as the foods I ate while I was actively dieting and now while I am maintaining my weight. As I said, it is

TABLE 6

My Diet

	OVERWEIGHT	DIETING	MAINTENANCE
6:00 AM	Bagel/Jelly	English muffin Jelly Egg whites (3)	English muffin Jelly Egg whites (3) Peanut butter
8:30 AM	Pastry	Nothing	Nothing
12:00 noon	Sandwich (½) Veggie sticks	Nonfat yogurt String cheese	Nonfat yogurt String cheese
4:00 PM	Snicker bar	Nothing	Balance Bar
7:00 PM	Meat/fish/fowl Rice Salad or vegetable 1-2 glass red wine	Meat/fish/fowl Vegetables Salad ½ glass red wine	Meat/fish/fowl Vegetables Salad 1-2 glass red wine

in part a discovery process. There are foods I eat now that I never ate before. An excellent example is string cheese. My kids actually ate string cheese but I had never tried it. One day a friend who understood the principles of the Zone Diet had mentioned to me what a great compliment it was to yogurt. I found it interesting because I had been eating a yogurt and banana for lunch and found it very poor in curbing my hunger over a number of hours. By adding a stick of string cheese, my hunger was markedly less. I then got rid of the banana and added a second stick of string cheese and that was ideal. Finally, a member of my staff pointed out the differences in protein content between the various nonfat yogurts and I ultimately arrived at the combination of food that I eat for lunch today. This was a process that evolved over two years. I am sure you will find different foods in your experiments that ultimately are adopted into your routine meals.

At this point you should have a good idea of what you will eat at breakfast, lunch and dinner. You may want to write those foods down. If you are still uncertain what you might have with certain meals, go to the tables at the end of the book. Remember to make food choices you like so it will be easier to maintain a long-term approach to eating better.

As I look back on my previous diet and consider what I eat now, there are several prominent contrasts. When I had a significant obesity problem, I never ate protein at breakfast. I would often have to eat frequently during the morning because I would get hungry before lunch. I usually ate a fairly reasonable amount of protein at lunch. My end of the afternoon snack is far different and far better at keeping me from getting hungry until dinner. I have given up fruits that have high sugar content or are high in what is commonly referred to as the glycemic index. Those fruits such as oranges, tangerines, grapes, etc., raise your blood sugar levels quickly and it drops just as quickly. I have given up orange juice and other high sugar drinks. Finally, I eat considerably more vegetables than I ever did before. In summary, I eat more vegetables, I eat less starch and I make sure I eat some lean protein early in the day. I think all of these are good changes to anyone's diet. I know these changes have worked for me.

Chapter Ten
DOC, THIS IS NOT WORKING

The majority of people who read this book and follow its principles will be able to achieve weight loss. There are, however, patients who fail to lose weight and I have come to recognize certain patterns. Interestingly, people have asked me to write this book for over a year now, but I am glad that I waited until now to complete it. Over the last year I think I have gained enough experience that it has allowed me to be able to write this important chapter. Men and women, I believe, fail my diet for different reasons. For that reason, I am going to deal with the issue of men who fail to lose weight first, and then women.

The primary reason men fail to lose weight on my diet is that they simply are not following it. A major problem is usually motivation. Their spouse may think the diet is a great idea and may be preparing meals appropriate at home. When I counsel my male patients regarding the diet and its principles, I often ask, "Who does the cooking at home?" Commonly it is the wife and she usually will listen intently. What she cannot control is what her husband may eat outside of the home, or if he simply refuses to follow the *three rules*. No dietary program will work for anyone not motivated to follow it.

My parents struggled with how to help me lose weight until one day in seventh grade I decided I was fat. I then went on a weight loss program I designed with my mother and returned to a normal body size. My parents were concerned and loving but no dietary program they proposed was going to work until I decided that I needed to lose weight. It is no different for my patients. Nothing can replace motivation.

A second reason men fail in the *three rule* diet is they simply do not understand their food groups. When a patient fails to lose weight, I often will specifically ask them what they eat for breakfast, lunch and dinner. Not uncommonly, one of my male patients will tell me he eats cereal, orange juice and a banana for breakfast. I listen intently and then ask him, "Where's the protein in this breakfast?" The patient will think about it for a few seconds and then softly respond, "The cereal?" My male patients have a much poorer understanding of the make-up of their foods than my female patients. These patients will often respond to additional education. If you think you are in this category, consider visiting a dietitian who will work with you on the principles of the *three rule* diet.

My female patients as a rule tend to be more motivated and have a better understanding of the various food groups. Women start with the disadvantage of a slower rate of metabolism than men, and may also have something in their genetic code that makes them less able to give up stored fat calories. As I stated earlier in the book, women probably on average have a greater tendency to gain weight more than men at any given carbohydrate level in their diet. Whereas the average male can probably consume a 50% carbohydrate diet, the average female is more likely to consume on the order of 40%. That means that some females may need to achieve as low as 20-30% carbohydrate intake before they can lose weight.

For those motivated people having difficulty, you will have to do more pencil work. I propose you keep a food diary. Write down, for at least 2-3 days, everything that you eat. Then, analyze those foods for their calories and various components of carbohydrate, protein and fat. Once you have established what you are eating and the proportions are right, then consider further reducing the amount of carbohydrate in your diet. The goal is to take your carbohydrate level from maybe 40% down to 30%. Try getting rid of or markedly reducing your carbohydrate intake at lunch. Apply the no white at night rule to lunch. If that still is not adequate, try getting rid of your starch intake as well at breakfast. By incorporating these changes, you are moving your carbohydrate intake as a percentage of your total calories closer and closer to that of the Atkin's diet. By following the other principles, however, you will not increase your fat intake on an absolute basis.

Another important question — if the diet principles are not working for you, have you increased your exercise? Exercise has the benefit of boosting your metabolism and having you expend more calories. Remember the best way to achieve weight loss over time is a combination of diet and exercise. If you did not start an exercise program, at least consider a walking program. It should dramatically improve the efficiency of your diet program.

Finally, if you have an adequate exercise program and feel that you have reduced your carbohydrate intake as low as possible, I would strongly recommend that you consider seeking professional nutritional advice. I do have patients who I have worked with upwards to a year and they have failed to lose weight. Over the course of the last year I have had at least six intelligent, motivated women in my practice that I referred to an intensive nutritional counseling service. It is expensive and it is time consuming, but every patient was able to achieve considerable weight loss. Every patient has thanked me for referring him or her to the organization.

I would also suggest you ask your doctor to check your thyroid and see if there is any other reason why you have not been able to lose weight. The great majority of patients I see do not need this type of intensive counseling nor are they willing to put up with the time involved or the expense. There are, however, a few individuals who have extreme difficulty in losing weight and if following the principles and the modifications I have outlined above are not working, then I would strongly suggest you take your food diaries and get further counseling.

Chapter Eleven
A PAT ON THE BACK

I have counseled hundreds of patients regarding their diet. When I am actively following my patients and trying to help them lose weight, I often see them once a month. When those patients achieve success, which can be losing two, four or even ten pounds in a month, they often return and feel elated. If you are able to achieve success with these dietary guidelines, and many do, I am sorry that I am not going to be able to share in your happiness.

When patients leave the exam room from their follow-up appointments and have been able to achieve weight loss, I usually congratulate them in front of my nursing staff. My nursing staff, some of whom have also followed the diet with success, share in their happiness as well and congratulate them. Since I am not able to do this in person, I would greatly appreciate it if you would stand in front of a mirror at the end of every month that you lose weight, look yourself right in the eye, and say, "Great Job." Losing weight is not that hard once you understand the principles. It does, however, take motivation and commitment over time. Now you are fitting in the clothes you have not worn to work in a long time, feeling more energetic and having friends ask you, "How'd you do it?"

For my diabetic patients who are able to achieve weight loss, we give them the same kudos in the office. The diabetic patients who are able to stop their medications because of weight loss get a special recognition — they get a hug in front of all my staff. Those people, men and women, have dramatically reduced their risk of cardiovascular disease and overcome the additional hurdle of medications that make you gain weight. That is a real accomplishment.

So I regret that I will not be there to share in your joy, but your friends will be. Many of them will ask how you lost your weight and you can explain the principles to them as well. Be an example that motivation, exercise and diet can cure obesity.

Breakfast Choices

Whole Wheat Toast 1 pc.   with   Soy Nut Butter
Almond Butter
Peanut Butter
Turkey Bacon
Canadian Bacon
Egg Whites 2-3,
Eggs (3) w/ (1) yolk,
or Breakfast Ham

Oatmeal   with   Above
or
Almonds
or
Protein Powder

Non Fat Yogurt   with   String Cheese
1-2 Tubes

REMEMBER!

Orange juice, most cereals, pastries and donuts are high in sugar and low in protein. These foods will lead to recurrent hunger in 2-3 hours and are poor choices.

Worst Choice - NO Breakfast.

Lunch Choices

Salad	with	Lean Meat Fish Fowl
Cottage Cheese Low Fat	with	Apple or Pear
Non Fat Yogurt	with	String Cheese 1-2 Tubes
Sandwich (1 slice bread)	with	Lean Deli Meat
Soup	with	Low Fat Cheese or String Cheese
Vegetables	with	Lean Meat Fish Fowl

Worst Choice - NO Lunch.

Late Afternoon Snack Choices

Non Fat Yogurt
String Cheese
Beef
Turkey Jerky
Smoked Fish
Apple or Pear with String Cheese
Balance Bar with 40-30-30 Content Blend
Almonds, Peanuts, Cashews

Bad Choices:
Candy
Candy Bars
Cookies
Cake
Donuts

REMEMBER!
Drink plenty of water and plan ahead so you
do not have to choose from bad choices.

Dinner Choices

Lean protein - 3-6 oz.

Meat/fish/fowl

Serving size comparable to a chicken breast
or a small steak.

Non starchy vegetables - unlimited

Salad - unlimited

Try to favor low fat or no fat salad dressing

No White at Night - see next page

No White at Night

Starches and high starch vegetables to avoid at night include:

Beans - Navy, Red, Pinto, Lima, Refried

Bread of any type

Corn

Pasta

Peas

Potatoes - Red, White, Sweet

Rice - Brown or White

Squash - Acorn, Butternut

Bibliography

1. Sears, Barry Ph.D. *The Zone Diet*. Regan Books, 1995.

2. Center for Disease Control. National Center for Health Statistics. *Overweight Prevalence Statistics*, 1999.

3. Fontaine, K.R., D.T. Redden, C. Wang, A.O. Westfall, and D.B. Allison. Years of Life Lost Due to Obesity. *JAMA* 289:187-193, 2003.

4. Serdula, M.K., A.H. Mokdad, D.F. Williamson, D.A. Galuska, J.M. Mendlein, and G.W. Heath. Prevalence of Attempting Weight Loss and Strategies for Control ling Weight. *JAMA* 282:1353-1358, 1999.

5. Maskalyk, J. Southern Africa's Famine Far Worse Than Anticipated. *CMAJ*; 167:11-12, 2002

6. Irwin, M.C., Y. Yasui , C.M. Ulrich, D. Bowen et al. Effect of Exercise on Total and Intra-Abdominal Body Fat in Postmenopausal Women. *JAMA* 289:323-330, 2003.

7. Atkin, R.C. *Dr. Atkin's New Diet Revolution*. New York: Avon Books, 1992.

8. Ludwig, D.S. The Glycemic Index. *JAMA* 287:2414-2423, 2002.

9. Mokdad, A.H., E.S. Ford, B.A. Bowman et. al. Prevalence of Obesity, Diabetes, and Obesity — Related Health Risk Factors, 2001. *JAMA* 289:76-79, 2003.

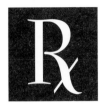

Exercise - walk one half hour per day

Eat three meals per day

Eat some lean protein with every meal

No white at night

Place this page on your refreigerator door.

Dr. Gavin's book available through:
Eld Inlet Publishing, LLC
2103 Harrison NW, Suite 2 - 316
Olympia, WA 98502-2607

Web Site: www.nowhiteatnight.com

To arrange a speaking engagement
by Dr. Gavin
call
(360) 413-8528

ORDER FORM

Name: _____

Address: _____

City: _____

State: _____ Zip: _____

Shipping Address: _____
No PO Boxes Please

Phone: ( ) _____ or ( ) _____

Qty	Price Each	Total
	$19.95 US	$
Sales Tax (WA residents only, add appropriate sales tax)		$
Shipping & Handling: (Call for information on larger shipments)		$ **FREE**
	TOTAL	$

Enclosed: ☐ Check ☐ Money Order for $ _____

☐ Visa ☐ MasterCard Exp. Date: _____

Credit Card #: _____

Signature: _____

Mail to: Eld Inlet Publishing, LLC
2103 Harrison NW, Suite 2 - 316, Olympia, WA 98502-2607
Phone: 360-866-9401